Green Tea
Healing Miracle

The Green Tea Report

Includes Latest Research on Cancer, Heart Disease, Arthritis, and More

Billie J. Sahley, Ph.D., C.N.C.
with
Katherine Birkner, C.R.N.A., Ph.D.

Pain & Stress Publications®
San Antonio, Texas
October 2006

Note to Readers

This material is not intended to replace services of a physician, nor is it meant to encourage diagnosis and treatment of illness, disease or other medical problems by the layman. This book should not be regarded as a substitute for professional medical treatment and while every care is taken to ensure the accuracy of the content, the authors and the publisher cannot accept legal responsibility for any problem arising out of experimentation with the methods described. Any application of the recommendations set forth in the following pages is at the reader's discretion and sole risk. If you are under a physician's care for any condition, he or she can advise you as to whether the programs described in this book are suitable for you.

This publication has been compiled through research resources at the **Pain & Stress Center**, San Antonio, Texas 78229.

October 2006
Printed in U.S.A

A Pain & Stress Publication®

Additional Copies Available from

Pain & Stress Center

5282 Medical Drive, Suite 160
San Antonio, TX 78229

1-800-669-2256

Library of Congress Number 2006933523

ISBN 978-1-889391-32-8

Acknowledgements

A special thanks to Scott Smith and staff of Taiyo International for all of your important research that you provided for this book.

Taiyo International for your support and for sharing your photos.

Barbara Garrett of Emory University for providing research information

Linda Volpenhein and Laura Boone for their many hours of proofing and editing.

The staff of the Pain & Stress Center for all their support and hard work to allow us the time to do needed research for this book.

Dedication

To my sister, Gloria Cavanaugh.

To the Lord for always lighting our paths.

Table of Contents

Foreword

Why did I decide to write this book on green tea?

This book is an answer to the hundreds of calls, emails, and letters we received asking us about the benefits of this healing nutrient, green tea. As I began to review all of the research on green tea, I found it hard to believe that this one nutrient had all of the healing and protective benefits. Green tea is thousands of years old and will certainly hold its place as a truly special nutrient.

As a health care practitioner, I have seen my patients suffer from a long list of illnesses. I found if they use preventative medicine, they are in a much better place and do not get sick as often, or are able to bounce back more quickly from an illness. So far green tea has been a godsend to everyone that has used it.

As I reviewed all of this information and

the clinical studies that are ongoing, I knew this book had to be written so I could share all of the information with you. Green tea extract will improve your life and protect you in so many ways as it has me and I know it will continue to. Thanks to studies being published each month, we have a constant support of all the information in this book! One of my major goals is to write books to keep you informed so you and your family can live a better quality of life naturally as we were meant to.

Dr. Billie J. Sahley

Green Tea
A Brief History

According to Chinese legend, green tea was discovered in 2737 B.C. Emperor Shen-Nung, a divine healer, always boiled his water before drinking. He noted that people who boiled water experienced longevity and better health. One afternoon he was boiling his water when some leaves from a nearby tree accidentally fell into his water. He liked the pleasant aroma so he took a sip; tea was born. He proclaimed it "heaven sent."

After water, tea is the most popular drink consumed in the world today. Since Shen-Nung discovered tea, tea has spread to Japan and the remainder of the Far East. Tea was brought to Europe by the Dutch and finally to America in 1650. The East India Company brought tea leaves to England in 1669. At first tea was very expensive and only the upper class could afford to purchase it. The cost at the time was about $30 to

$49 per pound. A pound of tea yields about two hundred tea bags. In the 1800s, ships brought tea from China to London and other parts of the world. Introduction of the speedy clipper ships expedited the trip to London and the supply increased so that it was not so expensive.

Green tea is made from the dried leaves of camellia sinensis, a perennial evergreen

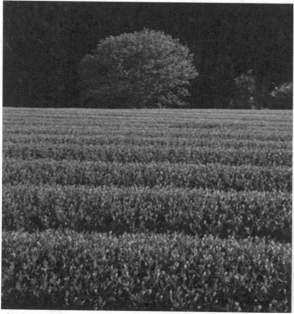

Cultivated green tea plants vs. standardized tea tree in Japan. (Courtesy of Taiyo International)

shrub. The medicinal healer has been used for 5,000 years. The tea plant, native to Southeast Asia, spontaneously grows from the tropics to the more temperate areas of Asia. Although it can reach heights of forty feet, most tea plants are maintained by pruning to two to three feet. The tea plant grows in more than 20 countries of Asia, Africa, and South America. Green tea, black tea and oolong tea all derive from the same plant. The number one producer of tea today is India followed by China, Kenya, Indonesia, Sir Lanka, and Japan. Of all the tea produced, the Japanese use 98% of the crop and the U.S. uses more than 80% of the remainder. Green tea in the U.S. is in demand and consumed daily by millions of people.

Green tea is a source of caffeine, a methylxanthine that stimulates the central nervous system, relaxes smooth muscles in the airway to the lungs, stimulates the heart increasing heart rate and blood pressure, and acts on the kidney as a diuretic increasing urine output. One cup of tea contains approximately 50 mgs of caffeine. Caffeine may cause insomnia if you ingest too much.

In addition caffeine may increase the production of stomach acid that aggravates ulcer symptoms. If you do not want the caffeine use decaf green tea extract that offers the same protection without the caffeine. Green tea contains polyphenols, catechins, anthocyanins, phenolic acids, tannin and trace elements of vitamins. The amount of caffeine, polyphenols, and theanine in the leaves of tea (C. Sinesis) determine the taste of tea.

Other components of green tea catechins are flavonoids, a strong antioxidant that trap and destroy free radicals. Vitamins B, C, and E are all found in green tea. Other important free radical fighting vitamins include:

Vitamin E, known to protect the heart, is a powerful antioxidant that slows the aging process.

Vitamin B aids in the metabolism of carbohydrates.

Vitamin C is a strong immune enhancer and fluoride, your mouth and teeth's best friend.

Green tea also contains amino acids.

Amino Acids Found in Green Tea Infusion

Theanine	45.0%
Glutamic acid	12.7%
Aspartic acid	10.8%
Arginine	9.2%
Glutamine	7.5%
Serine	3.8%
Threonine	1.4%
Alanine	1.4%
Asparagine	1.2%
Lysine	1.0%
Phenylalanine	1.1%
Valine	1.0%

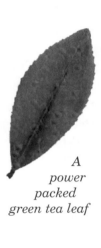

A power packed green tea leaf

Fermentation is the most important process in tea manufacturing for consumption. Enzymes present in the leaves of tea are responsible for the conversion of tannin. The amount of fermentation significantly affects the type and quality of tea. Tea is classified according to the amount of fermentation; green tea is unfermented, oolong undergoes semi-fermentation while black tea is fully fermented.

The main free radical fighter is EGCG. Green tea leaves are steamed to prevent oxidation of EGCG compound so they remain potent. The steaming occurs immediately after harvesting to inactivate the enzymes that lower the EGCG potency. Records show tea has a track record of 5,000 years and the Chinese emperor Shen-Nung who was a divine healer deserves the credit for discovering this healing nutrient. The monks began using it for various medical purposes and word spread about the benefits and its healing power. Tea has a long record of how it made its way through China and other countries to end up in the United States as a healing wonder. Now that you have an idea of how all of this came about, let's examine all of the healing wonders of green tea and the research that supports all its healing magic. In the next few years, green tea will take a major step in the information regarding natural medicine.

Healing Properties of Green Tea

The healing properties of Green Tea Extract offer a promise of healing that no other nutritional supplement can. The documented research behind this biochemical superstar has described Green Tea as *possibly the most potent natural anti-cancer nutrient ever discovered.* Numerous volumes of scientific research document the multiple benefits of green tea. The most important studies prove that green tea does inhibit the development of undesirable cell colonies and suppress the proliferation of existing cell colonies. Green tea protects against experimentally induced DNA damage by stopping the progression of undesirable cell colonies. Green tea works as a cancer fighter with its unique ability to block a protein that is involved in the growth of tumor cells. Research now in progress at University of Rochester in New York found the chemical in green tea that binds to a protein called HSP90 is present at elevated levels in cancer cells. Green tea EGCG (Epigallocatechin Gallate) binds to the HSP90 and prevents from cell receptor activation that plays a role in turning on harmful genes. EGCG is the main active component (polyphenols) of green tea that has the highest concentration of catechins. EGCG potent antioxidant polyphenols are at least 300 to 400 times more active than Vitamin C and 25 times more effective than Vitamin E at shielding cells and their DNA from free radical damage. Scientists believe damage to the cells and DNA is the link to heart disease, cancer, and other illnesses. Catechins reduce the occurrence of cancer. EGCG reduces oxidation of active oxygen from free radicals, lowers blood cholesterol, improves cardiovascular health and atherosclerosis (thickening, hardening, and lack of elasticity of arteries). Catechins inhibit blood pressure and blood sugar increases. Catechins kill bacteria and viruses and fight carcinogenic bacteria. Catechins are very powerful disease fighters and potent antioxidants that have multiple beneficial effects.

As far back as 1965 medical researchers reported people who consumed Chinese green tea have a greater protection against cancer and a much stronger immune system. Continued research uncovered more information about lower cancer rates in China and Japan as well as longevity among the Asian population. As research continued in green tea scientists found that one of the major components was EGCG. EGCG behaves much like methotrexate, an antimetabolite used in the treatment of breast, head, neck, lungs, blood, bone, lymphatic system, and uterine cancer. EGCG has the highest level and broadest spectrum of cancer fighting activity. The most important factor in cancer treatment and prevention are the polyphenols in green tea and green tea extract. Of all the different polyphenols, EGCG (epigallocatechin gallate) stands above the rest. EGCG is a powerful antioxidant that is an important player in the therapeutic properties of green tea. Scientists believe that green tea works by inhibiting cell replication and enzymes that prevent cancer growth as well as other cellular processes.

A study conducted at Harvard Medical School demonstrated that 20 genes are critical for learning. But deterioration may begin as early as age 40. Research reveals these genes are also involved in the memory and plasticity of brain function. The brain tissue studied was from 30 individuals ages 26 to 98. Samples from individuals aged 71 plus years all had similar amounts of deterioration in the brain. Test results showed deterioration levels of those ages of 40 to 70 varied greatly. The results demonstrated there was not a consistent amount of deterioration that seemed to progress with age. Results reflected that some individuals in their 40's had very high levels of gene deterioration, while some individuals in their 60's had relatively low levels of deterioration. The group that used supplements containing antioxidants on a regular basis showed the lowest amount of deterioration. The Harvard research group believes exposure to free radicals and toxins might be the cause of premature damage. Researchers suggest lifestyle changes should included exercise, stress reduction and consumption of foods high in antioxidants, specifically green tea extract supplements. Clinical data reflects green tea supplements help people with depressed immune systems in as little as two weeks.

Teas contain antioxidants called polyphenols. Several types of polyphenols include thearubigins, theaflavins, catechins, flavonols, hydroxycinnamates, and gallic acid. High levels of the powerful antioxidants in green tea extract help protect the brain from damage done by free radicals. Free radicals act as an aggressive accelerator of the aging process to tissue and brain cells. The damage of free radicals threatens the overall health of the brain's learning and memory function as early as age 40. Free radicals cause damage to the tissue cells of all organs in the body, heart, lungs, stomach, and brain. Green tea protects the organs and guards against heart disease by lowering cholesterol. The *Journal of the American College of Surgeons* (May 2006) reported researchers at Yale University detailed the body of evidence linking green tea to better heart health and a lower risk of cancer.

Nutritional medicine practitioners suggest you give strong consideration to taking two green tea extract supplements (at least 1,000 mg) on a daily basis. Cancer researchers have established that green tea can block the production of urokinase, which basically works as fuel for growing tumors. This natural miracle can slow aging of the skin and kills bacteria that cause bad breath, tooth decay, and gingivitis. The decaffeinated green tea extract used by the Pain & Stress Center was selected for its premium quality and gentle processing methods. This preserved the precious antioxidants known as polyphenols; water-soluble compounds that make up a subgroup of flavonoids.

A 2003 study in cancer research demonstrates a strong link between anti-cancer activities and their inhibition of critical pathways necessary for the development of many common malignancies. Polyphenols comprise approximately 30 percent of the green tea leaf; the primary polyphenol is the very potent and popular Epigallocatechin Gallate (EGCG.) One cup of green tea contains 150 milligrams of EGCG and a total of 275 mgs. of catechins. Recently many researchers have focused on the preventive effect on adult disease using green tea polyphenols and decaffeinated green tea polyphenols and purified compounds.

Well-controlled clinical trials have shown that green tea helps prevent cancer of the pancreas, colon, small intestine, stomach, breast, and lung. *No other supplement can make this claim.* Increasing evidence supports that green tea helps prevent skin cancer and studies support that it induces death in human prostate cancer cells. Not one but two miracles come from green tea. Theanine, the major amino acid found in green tea, has been found to have beneficial effects by raising the levels of serotonin and dopamine in specific areas of important brain regions, particularly the hypothalamus, hippocampus (the brain's memory center), and the striatum. You can use Theanine on a daily basis for stress, anxiety, or PMS. Studies reflect theanine increases alpha waves in the brain. When the brain waves are in the alpha state, it indicates a deep state of relaxation or meditation. Concentration enhances and the alpha waves cause muscle relaxation that decreases stress-tension and pain. Theanine is a major neurotransmitter in the brain and enhances brain functions. The effects of theanine are felt the same day you take it. I have found theanine to be one of the best natural sources to reduce stress and anxiety. Make sure the green tea is Suntheanine. Suntheanine is the trade name for Taiyo International's patented pure form L-Theanine.

Americans should take a lesson from the Japanese. Sit back, relax, and drink a cup of green tea with two theanine. Theanine has the ability to increase GABA and other inhibitory neurotransmitters such as the feel good chemical, dopamine in the brain. Theanine gives you the control feeling you enjoy without the anxiety. For more in depth information, read my book, *Theanine, The Relaxation Amino Acid.*

Dr. Stephen Hsu, cell biologist and cancer researcher, has been very interested in the properties of green tea. He observed that populations that drink green tea regularly have much lower cancer rates than those who don't. His research helped determine that green tea polyphenols helped eliminate free radicals that damage DNA and lead to cancer. After extensive research, Dr. Hsu found green tea induced p57, a protein that regulates cell growth and differentiates changes in the behavior of healthy cells as polyphenols target cancer cells for destruction. This change in behavior protects the healthy cells.

The *National Cancer Institute* awarded Dr. Hsu a grant for research comparing healthy cells to cancer cells after exposure to compounds in green tea called polyphenols. The *Cancer Institute* grant will help Dr. Hsu determine the exact cellular and genetic behavior involved in the p57 process. The grant funding helps establish researchers and further refine their understanding of how green tea polyphenols both protect healthy cells and declare war on cancer cells. In 1994, the *Journal of the National Cancer Institute* published an epidemiological study indicating drinking green tea reduced the risk of esophageal cancer in Chinese men and women by 60%. University of Purdue researchers concluded the compound in green tea inhibits the growth of cancer cells and also lowers cholesterol as well as improving the ratio of good HDL cholesterol to bad LDL cholesterol. Continued research demonstrated the following health conditions improve with the intake of green tea: cancer, rheumatoid arthritis, high cholesterol level, cardiovascular disease, infection, and impaired immune function. Another study at Vanderbilt University reported theaflavins-enriched green tea extract lowers cholesterol.

Studies done at several universities show catechins possess diverse pharmacological properties that include anti-carcinogenic, anti-arteriorsclerotic, and antibacterial effects. Catechins reduce the evidence of cancer, reduce oxidation by active oxygen, and lower blood cholesterol. Catechins also inhibit the increase of blood pressure, and blood sugar. Catechins kill bacteria and viruses and fight carcinogenic bacteria. Catechins are very powerful disease fighters and potent antioxidants that have multiple beneficial effects.

The most important factor in cancer

treatment and prevention are the polyphenols in green tea extract that have the highest amount of this important chemical.

Types of Catechins

Catechin (C)
Epicatechin (EC)
Gallocatechin (GC)
Epigallocatechin (EGC)
Epicatechin gallate (ECg)
Epigallocatechin gallate (EGCG or EGCg)

Of all the polyphenols, one stands above the rest, EGCg (or EGCG). EGCG (Epigallocatechin Gallate) is a very powerful antioxidant that is a vital player in the therapeutic properties of green tea. Scientists believe it works by inhibiting cell replication and enzymes that prevent cancer growth as well as other cellular processes.

You should take at least 1,000 to 2,000 milligrams of green tea extract daily to gain the protection and health benefits. Make sure it is decaffeinated and pure green tea extract. Thus far, scientists are impressed with the research that supports green tea and documents its effectiveness to fight and prevent breast cancer. The results of their work was published in the December issue of *Cancer Research*, the official journal of the American Cancer Association for Cancer Research. New research supports a powerful antioxidant known as EGCG. EGCG binds to a protein found on tumor cell, thus slowing or destroying the cells before it develops. The progression of cancer research in all areas is growing every day as a positive way to stop the dreaded disease and is pointing scientists in the right direction. Researchers found that EGCG, a compound in green tea, inhibits an enzyme required for cancer cell growth and kills cancer cells with no ill effect on healthy cells.

Researchers have found an ingredient that kills cancer cells while sparing healthy cells. Hasan Mukhtar, a professor of dermatology at Case Western Reserve University (CWRU), tested the ingredient EGCG on cancerous human cells of the skin, lymph system, prostate, and on normal human cells in mice. Green Tea's polyphenols pack 300 to 400 times the antioxidant power of Vitamins

E and C, says lead study author Tariq M. Haqqi, Ph.D., from Case Western Reserve University in Cleveland. Polyphenols seem to slam the door on dangerous inflammatory cells that migrate into joints and do the most rheumatoid arthritis damage. Early test tube studies hint that green tea may stop the destruction of human cartilage cells caused by osteoarthritis.

Throughout China and Japan, green tea is part of their regular diet, especially among senior citizens. Numerous epidemiological research studies consistently documents green tea consumption with a lower frequency of cancers. In 1989 clinical study in the *Japanese Journal of Nutrition* reported that specific areas and regions of Japan where residents consume green tea in multiple forms has a much lower death rate from stomach cancer than other regions of Japan. Green tea is a rising star. In 1994 a clinical study report reflected how green tea protected smokers. In 1994 the *Journal of the National Cancer Institute* reported a case control study conducted at the Shanghai Cancer Institute in China.

The results demonstrated that tea drinkers had a 50% reduction in the risk for esophageal and stomach cancers. The May 1998 *Oncology Report* disclosed that when human stomach cancers were exposed to green tea extract and EGCG (a major component of the extract) both inhibited cell growth and induced apoptosis (cell death). The researchers suggest that consuming green tea in large amounts possibly protects humans from stomach cancer.

A report in *Biochemistry* (Vol. 44, April 2005) about a study conducted at the University of Rochester Medical Center in New York found a potential new mechanism of action for green tea and its active compounds against cancer. Green tea protects against cancer by having an effect on a wandering protein. Drug industry researchers are already targeting the research on anti-cancer drugs. This protein would probably respond to the EGCG in green tea, so cancer would be stopped in its tracks. Reports in the *Chemistry and Application of Green Tea* show that green tea polyphenols clearly have anti-tumor activities in various organs.

NIH also evidenced the effect of green tea polyphenols on colon cancer, and in the last five years the U.S. government has funded more than 150 studies on green tea and its constituent chemicals. Green tea's antioxidants disrupt the chemical pathways inside cancer cells by gobbling up free radicals.

Green Tea and Medical Conditions

American Cancer Society

Tea plays a possible role in preventing some types of cancer according to researcher, Dr. John Weisburger. He presented his report at the Second International Scientific Symposium on Tea and Human Health in Washington, D.C. Dr. Weisburger stated "The antioxidants in tea prevent the formation hazardous product that occur in the body during normal metabolic reactions. The antioxidants in tea lower the formation of these dangerous, oxidized forms of chemicals that may cause cancer in the human body". Defective cells are supposed to "apoptosis" (i.e., commit cell suicide). Cancer starts to become a threat to the body when defective cells keep right on growing and dividing, so failure of the cell death program is one of the hallmarks of cancer. The Indian Institute of Technology in Kharagpur, West Bengal India studied the effect of green tea polyphenols, especially the catechins, on the development of blood vessels (angiogenesis) in tumors. The results show that green tea catechins reduce the vascularization of blood vessels. The green tea polyphenols inhibit the proliferation and migration of endothelial cells and strongly inhibit the formation of new blood vessels in tumors and atherosclerosis lesions to advanced plaques. The new blood vessels supply oxygen and nutrients to the surrounding tissues. This hinders tumor progression and may explain the beneficial effect on coronary heart disease and cancer.

Every person suffering from cancer, at risk for being diagnosed with cancer, or having a family history of cancer, should take green tea extract supplements. Green tea supplements have no negative side effects, yet provide powerful anticancer and antioxidant compounds.

Prostate Cancer and Green Tea

Prostate cancer is the number one cancer for non-smoking American men and African American men are two and one half times more likely to develop prostate cancer. Prostate cancer is mainly a disease of aging. Men can develop prostate cancer in their thirties and forties, but it occurs increasingly in men after the age of 55. About 80% of all cases occur in men over 65 years of age, which increases to 80% by age 80. An Italian study of 32 men took a look at green tea ingredients to decrease the risk of prostate cancer in men at high risk for developing prostate cancer. The men selected to participate in the study had high grade PINS (prostatic intraepithelial neoplasms), a precursor to prostate cancer. The men were divided into two groups randomly. One group took 200 mg of green tea preparation three times daily while the other group took a placebo for a year. One man developed cancer in the group that took 600 mg of green tea preparation daily whereas nine developed cancer in the group taking a placebo. The study found that a man would have to drink 12 to 15 cups of tea per day to equal the amount of catechins. Research established that the polyphenols in green tea boosts the number of enzymes that convert carcinogens in the prostate to harmless inactive chemicals.

The Mayo Clinic study, published in the August 1998 issue of the *Journal Cancer Letter,* found that green tea not only inhibited cell growth, it also produced fragmented nuclei and other signs of apoptosis, or programmed cell death. Since prostate cancer has a long latency period and usually does not develop until the mid-fifties, it is best to prevent prostate cancer through chemoprevention using green tea. Research shows that green tea polyphenols such as epigallocatechin-3-gallate, epigallocatechin, and epicatechins-3-gallate when given to TRAMP (transgenic mouse model that copies the progressive forms of human prostate cancer) demonstrated remarkable preventative effects against the development of prostate cancer.

Green Tea and Ovarian Cancer

Epidemiological laboratory studies indicate that green and black tea may protect against various cancers. A study from Sweden took a look at tea consumption and the risk of ovarian cancer in 61,057 women aged 40 to 76 years of age. The women competed a 67 item food frequency study between 1987 to 1990 with cancer follow-up through December 2004. In the fifteen years, 301 women developed invasive epithelial ovarian cancer. The risk of ovarian cancer was inversely associated with tea consumption from none or seldom to less than one cup daily; 1 cup per day; and 2 or more cups per day. Every additional cup decreased the incidence of cancer by 18%. The researchers concluded that ovarian cancer decreases with tea consumption in a dose-dependent manner.

Green Tea and Gastritis

An epidemiological study at Kuwait University suggest that high consumption of green tea guards against the development of chronic gastritis and reduces the risk of stomach cancer. Part of the study looked at the effect of green tea, black tea, and Vitamin E on intestinal mucosa. Green tea helped protect the intestines from damage before a fast and reversed atrophy that was induced by fasting. Black tea had no effect while Vitamin E protected to a lesser degree. Another study done in China and published in the *International Journal of Cancer* found that drinking tea decreases the risk of biliary tract cancers and biliary stones (gallbladder and bile ducts), especially in women. Although these cancers are rare, they are highly fatal cancers. Ingestion of at least 1 cup of green tea daily could decrease the risk of gallbladder and bile duct cancers by 40%. Dr. Hsing of NIH concluded, "The exact mechanism by which the tea can protect against biliary tract cancers are unclear, but may involve antiproliferative and anti-inflammatory properties of tea polyphenols, in particular epigallocatechin-3-gallate (EGCG)." Drinking green tea is protective against a variety of cancers including gastrointestinal. Most ingested polyphenols concentrate in the gastrointestinal tract and are not well absorbed into the remainder of the body. When green tea polyphenols are present in high concentrations in the gut, the therapeutic potential is very high. Polyphenols are a major source of antioxidants, but also are antiviral, antibacterial, anti-inflammatory, and anticarcinogenic. Green tea polyphenols are effective in inflammatory bowel disease. While esophageal cancer prevention studies are inconsistent, cancers of the stomach and colon are inversely proportionate to amount of tea consumed. Simply put, green tea acts as a preventative for stomach and colon cancers.

Pancreatic cancer is the fifth leading cause of cancer deaths in the U.S. and the five-year survival rate is 4%. The standard treatment for pancreatic cancer often yields poor outcomes even if diagnosed early. In the *International Journal of Gastrointestinal Cancer*, M. W. Roomi, et. al, suggest the combination of green tea extract, lysine, proline, and ascorbic acid (Vitamin C) offers promise as an adjunct to standard treatment of pancreatic cancer. Another study from Kobe University School of Medicine in Kobe, Japan demonstrated that EGCG from green tea consumption lowered the risk of several human cancers. The study looked at pancreatic cancer cells and EGCG. EGCG significantly reduced the growth of pancreatic cells in a dose dependent manner and suppressed invasive ability of the cancer cells. In 1999 *Nutrition and Cancer* journal explored the chemopreventative effects of tea extracts, polyphenols, and EGCG on human pancreatic and prostate tumors in vitro. The results showed that tea extracts significantly inhibited cell growth. The study suggests that components of green tea can modulate the expression of genes known to play a role in cancer and potential agents in chemoprevention against pancreatic cancer. A case control study looked at cancer of the pancreas. Seventy-one patients were matched on sex and age (+ or – 3 years) to 142 community-based controls. All of the patients were questioned about demographic factors, diet, beverage consumption, and medical history. Consumption of raw vegetables and green tea considerably decreased risks, while consumption of meat with fat, boiled fish, coffee, black tea, and alcoholic beverages increased risks significantly.

Dr. Nicholas Gonzales received a grant from NIH to study an alternative treatment for pancreatic cancer. The clinical trials began stage III phase. Dr. Gonzalez's protocol involves dietary changes with detoxification using daily coffee enemas, pancreatic enzymes, and dietary supplements. The survival rate of his patients was three times that of traditional cancer treatments.

As you age you do not produce enough enzymes and begin to have digestive problems. Many people complain of indigestion or stomach problems after eating. They complain of gas, bloating, and belching. Gas results when you cannot digest the foods that you eat. Nutrients important to digestion include Super Pancreatin and glutamine. Pancreatin is a digestive enzyme that helps break down foods for uptake in the intestine. Super Pancreatin was formulated to address the specific digestive enzyme deficiencies. Add two pancreatin to each meal to aid digestion of your foods. Glutamine is vital for intestinal health. Glutamine assists your intestines, colon, and stomach in healing if you have had problems with digestion. You can use glutamine at any age, newborn to 100; it is a safe amino acid. Pure glutamine powder dissolves readily in water or juice and is tasteless. Heat destroys glutamine so do not add to a hot beverage.

Green Tea and Colon Cancer

Colon cancer is the third most common cancer found in men and women in the U.S. Colon and rectal cancers grow gradually over an interval of several years. Most colon cancers begin as polyp or a growth of tissue into the center of the colon or rectum. Over time the polyp can become cancerous and 95% of the time is an adenoma. But removing the polyp early when it first forms may prevent it from becoming cancerous.

A study in China examined the benefits of green tea and cancer. The study looked at 931 colon cancer patients, 884 rectum cancers, 451 pancreatic cancers, and 1552 controls. The patients with largest consumption of green tea has the strongest trends, especially with rectal and pancreatic cancers. The research findings give further evidence that drinking green tea may lower the risk of colorectal and pancreatic cancers.

Green Tea and Bladder Cancer

Bladder cancer is the fourth most common cancer in men and the tenth among women. Bladder cancer often reoccurs even when treated and prognosis is poor once it metastasizes. A preliminary study published in the *International Journal of Urology* of human bladder cell cancers showed that a combination of green tea extract, ascorbic acid (Vitamin C), lysine, proline, and arginine significantly reduced the invasion of human bladder cancer cells. The authors concluded that this combination is an excellent candidate for therapeutic treatment of bladder cancer by inhibiting the cancer development and spread. Another study conducted at UCLA and published in the *Clinical Cancer Research* journal on the effect of green tea and bladder cancer cells. An initial study using test tubes found green tea extract targeted cancer cells without harming the healthy cells. Other studies established that green tea extract induced death to cancer cells by cutting off the essential blood supply preventing development and spread. The study involved former smokers with bladder cancer to see if green tea extract prevented reoccurrence. The UCLA study continues.

More Evidence on Green Tea

A new study by a team of Swedish researchers adds support to the growing body of evidence that green tea contains compounds that fight cancer. Dr. Yihai Cao and Dr. Renhai Cao of the Karolinski Institute of Stockholm found that green tea contains EGCG that inhibits blood vessel growth. By preventing new blood vessel formation, it would not allow the tumor to survive or grow. Other studies show EGCG blocks an enzyme needed for cancer cell growth and kept cells from becoming cancerous without harming surrounding cells.

Green Tea and Breast Cancer

In a paper delivered at the ASCB (American Society of Cell Biology), scientists reported that green tea affects an enzyme known as NOX. According to these scientists, normal cells express the NOX enzyme only when they are dividing in response to growth hormone signals. In contrast, cancer cells have somehow gained the ability to express NOX activity at all times. This tumor-associated NOX activity is call tNOX. These scientists found that a substance in green tea—epigallocatechin gallate, or EGCG for short—interfered with tNOX, but not with normal NOX. This was the first study to directly link the EGCG in green tea to anticancer activity. In the laboratory, EGCG limited the activity of breast cancer tumor cells but did not affect normal, healthy breast cells. This might be one explanation as to why the incidence of breast cancer is so low in countries like Japan where green tea is consumed daily.

Researchers at Purdue University found that EGCG (epigallocatechin gallate) hinders an enzyme needed for cancer cell growth and kills cancer cells without any ill effects to healthy cells. The Purdue researchers established how cancer cells die. The cancer cells in the presence of EGCG fail to grow after division because the cells do not reach the minimum size needed to divide. They underwent programmed cell death or apoptosis.

Another study at UCLA demonstrated that green tea extract inhibits breast cancer growth by direct anti-proliferative effect on the cancer cells plus indirectly by suppression of the cancer cells. The study looked at the simultaneous administration of green tea to the standard breast cancer therapy. Green tea increases the inhibitory effect of tamoxifen on the growth of the estrogen-receptor positive human breast cancer cells in vitro. The combination was more effective at increasing cell death than either agent alone. Green tea decreased estrogen-receptor levels in cancer cells. The combination of green tea and tamoxifen suppresses cancer cell growth and may lead to future improvements in the treatment and prevention of breast cancer.

Green Tea, Tooth Decay, and Oral Cancer

Research explored green tea as prevention of tooth decay and oral cancer. The study looked at the effect of green and black tea leaves for delivery of catechins and theaflavins to the mouth. The subjects held green tea leaves (2 g) or brewed black tea (2 g of black leaves in 100 ml) in the mouth for 2 to 5 minutes. After rinsing the mouth thoroughly, the concentrations of catechins and theaflavins were measured in the saliva. High concentrations of both catechins and theaflavins were seen after the first hour. Researchers concluded that tealeaves provided a slow release source of catechins and theaflavins for potential prevention of oral cancer and tooth decay. Other researchers confirm that green tea does prevent dental caries.

Green Tea and Leukemia

Doctors at Mayo Clinic discovered that three of four patients with leukemia who ingested green tea or taking green tea extracts had signs of regression. The fourth had improvement in her white blood cell count, but her leukemia remained unchanged. The patients had chronic lymphocytic leukemia (CLL), a cancer involving white blood cells and bone marrow. CLL typically occurs during or after middle age and progresses slowly often over years.

Another patient had progressive swelling in her lymph nodes. She began taking green tea capsules twice daily and over the next year, her lymph nodes progressively shrank in size. One woman who had been diagnosed with CLL over five years ago began using a green tea patch applied to the skin. The patch provided 300 mg of polyphenols daily. In additions, she drank three cups of green tea daily that contained 300 mg polyphenols. After one month she stopped the patches, but continued to consume the green tea daily. After 15 months of daily green tea consumption laboratory tests confirmed her improvement and that her CLL had not progressed.

Green Tea, Smoking, and Lung Cancer

Researchers at Britain's Rochester University found that two chemicals in green tea shut down one of the major means that tobacco uses to trigger cancer. Drinking tea or supplementing with green tea extract may lower your risk considerably of developing lung cancer, even if you smoke.

Dr. Bouer E. Sumpio and his colleagues at Yale University School of Medicine released research that indicates green tea has a high concentration of antioxidants and catechins offering a range of health benefits. The key is in the antioxidants that help quench molecules known as oxygen free radicals. When there is an excess of free radicals they can damage body cells and potentially lead to disease. Tobacco smoke contains a large amount of free radicals. Although many Asian men smoke heavily, the rate of lung cancer is low compared to the U.S. Researchers attribute the lower cancer rate to green tea consumption due to its antioxidant properties.

Coronary heart disease (CHD) begins with an overload of free radicals and then arteries feeding the heart become hardened. This results in the arteries narrowing due to a buildup of plaques that are full of cholesterol forms on the artery walls. Dr. Sumpio and his research team report that green tea catechins—especially EGCG—could help the CHD process.

Green Tea and Diabetes

Diabetes is a disease characterized by the insufficient secretion or malfunction of insulin. Insulin regulates the amount of sugar in body tissues. Improper absorption of sugar causes excess concentrations in the blood. The body tries to lower blood sugar by excreting it through the kidneys via urine. Improper diet and sugar abuse usually leads to other immune problems. Research documents green tea polyphenol catechins lower blood sugar.

Blood sugar increases with age, accelerating aging by cross-linking with protein. Green tea lowers serum glucose. Green tea catechins (EGCG) enhance the action of insulin. This information was reported by the U.S. Department of Agriculture. Further research found EGCG influences the primary way glucose is absorbed in the blood. EGCG may help diabetics by mimicking the actions of insulin and inhibiting the liver's production of glucose, thereby lowering blood sugar. Continued research suggests green tea catechins can reduce the amount of glucose that passes through the intestine into the blood. Suggested dose is 2,000 milligrams of green tea extract daily.

The second part of the diabetes story concerns the pre-diabetic condition, Metabolic Syndrome or Syndrome X. The group most affected by this problem is one-third of middle-aged Americans who are not even aware they have a problem. *Forbes Magazine* (August 6, 2001) ran a story stating Syndrome X is the variable combination of obesity, high blood cholesterol, and hypertension linked by underlying resistance to insulin. Stephen Holt, M.D. has written an excellent book on Syndrome X entitled *Combat Syndrome X, Y and Z*. If you have Metabolic Syndrome you are in a class that is headed for diabetes and cardiovascular disease, which often accompanies diabetes. Metabolic Syndrome promotes a form of obesity most strongly linked to degenerative disease and a future of extreme pain and multiple limitations. Green tea does have the ability to suppress your blood sugar levels and enhance insulin function. Green tea extract stimulates the use of fatty acids by the muscle, reduces carbohydrate use, and allows longer exercise periods. Green tea enhances amylase, an enzyme that reduces glucose molecules so they can be absorbed into the bloodstream and used as fuel. Research demonstrates green tea assists the body to remove excess fat. Research will continue into the utilization of green tea therapy for diabetes to find all of the benefits that are available.

Insulin regulates the amount of sugar in body tissue. Improper absorption of sugar has been found to cause excess concentrations in the blood. When blood sugar levels increase over 160 mg/dL, the kidneys excrete excess sugar in an attempt to lower the blood sugar. Three signs of diabetes are polyphagia (excessive hunger that leads to increased food intake), polydipsia (excessive thirst), and polyuria (excessive urination). Improper diet and sugar abuse usually leads to other immune problems. Research documents that green tea polyphenols and catechins lower blood sugar. A report from the U.S. Department of Agriculture showed that green tea catechins (EGCG) enhance the action of insulin. Further research found

EGCG influences the primary way glucose is absorbed in the blood. It is possible that EGCG helps diabetics by mimicking the actions of glucose, thus lowering blood sugar. Continued research suggests green tea catechins reduce the amount of glucose that passes through the intestine into the blood. Suggested dose is 1,000 to 2,000 milligrams of green tea extract daily for blood sugar. A studied published in the *Annuals of Internal Medicine* (144, 8:554–556,2006), a high intake of green tea may inhibit the risk of Type 2 diabetes, and transdermal tea delivery may improve the bioavailability of

---

Metabolic Syndrome that has three or more of the following abnormalities:

Waist circumference greater than 40 inches in men and 35 inches in women

Serum triglyceride levels of 150 mg/dL or higher

Blood pressure of 130/85 or higher

Fasting blood glucose of 110 mg /dL or higher.

EGCG, the most studied catechin.

Metabolic syndrome X is the variable combination of obesity, high blood cholesterol and hypertension linked by underlying resistance to insulin. Metabolic syndrome increases your risk of developing heart disease, stroke, and diabetes due to the array of health factors. These risks increase your chance of succumbing to cardiovascular disease, stroke, and all causes. Green tea extract 1000 milligrams daily along with alpha lipoic acid, chromium picolinate, and vanadium helps keep blood sugar in the normal range. Follow a diet that is free of sugar. Utilizing the glycemic index foods helps prevent insulin and blood sugar spikes.

In the 2005 issue of *Textbook of Functional Medicine* green tea has an important effect on insulin modulation. Primary phytonutrients in green tea are the catechins and epicatechins. Catechins are insulin sensitizer and pancreatic protectants that are very helpful in the delay of glucose absorption and stops glucose production. In the USDA study researchers discussed other research including the anti-diabetic effect of tea on humans that is being investigated. In one clinical trial subjects ingested tea catechins 200 to 500 mg before ingesting 50 grams of starch. Starch, in most cases, converts to glucose by the digestive enzymes, mainly with alpha amylase. Glucose production was suppressed apparently because the catechins inhibit the enzyme actions. Other results demonstrate the green tea polyphenols remarkably suppress the uptake of glucose by the intestines for transfer into the bloodstream. The results showed the suppression is the strongest with the same catechins compounds that are the most active in enhancing insulin activity. Many researchers report green tea has a thermogenic effect in enhancing insulin activity. Many researchers report green tea has a thermogenic effect or fat burning ability; so if you want to lose a few pounds, this is great news.

Millions of women are in search of a way to maintain youthful skin. The answer is green tea. The major cause of skin aging is free radicals that everyone has in their bloodstream. Researchers found if you apply green tea extract to the skin topically, you can block the damage done by free radicals from ultraviolet B (UVB) light. Scientists found the topical application of green tea extract inhibits free radical activity. When measured in terms of lipid peroxidation, they had a 75 to 95% reduction and protein oxidation. When scientists measured skin aging damage, they found significant protective effects conferred by green tea. Scientists took the test one step further and added green tea extract to drinking water. They found much of the same results occurred, but comparatively less than when the green tea extract was applied topically. The skin directly absorbs the green tea extract, and then it goes into the bloodstream to perform its protective work. An article in the August 2005 issue of *Archives of Dermatology* stated there are benefits of green tea in human skin products. Green tea's antioxidant property is key to its skin protective qualities. Of all the antioxidants known, the components of green tea are the most potent. Antioxidants are agents that can counteract the effects of oxidant (free) radicals. Free radicals cause damage to cells and tissues. Antioxidants bind to free radicals deactivating them before they cause damage. Most of the polyphenols in green tea are catechins. Dr. Hasan Mukhtar, professor and director of research at Case Western Reserve University in Cleveland, reports that green tea catechins are antioxidants that are the most effective agent against skin inflammation and cancerous changes in the skin. In the June 2005 *Journal of the American Academy of Dermatology,* S. Hsu describes green tea catechins as chemopreventative, natural healing, and anti-aging agents for human skin.

Green Tea and Brain Health

Green tea protects against damage caused by heart attacks and strokes (brain accidents). Green teas' longevity extends to over 5,000 years. In the United Kingdom's *Journal of the Federal Experimental Biology,* research shows that green tea contains a chemical that reduces the amount of cell death that follows various traumas. When cell death occurs, it leads to tissue death that leads to organ failure. Further research demonstrates that green tea protects the brain from oxidative and chronic stress and anxiety as well as lowering monoamine oxidase (MAO) activity.

Research documents green tea protects the brain from oxidative stress, and lowers monoamine oxidase activity. Neurodegenerative diseases have been linked to both free radical damage and excessive breakdown of neurotransmitters caused by high monoamine oxidase activity. Studies have found that green tea and its phenolic components; catechins and epigallocatechin gallate are effective in inhibiting MAO and lowers peroxide levels in glial cells in the brain. Studies of the effects of catechins on nerve cell cultures show green tea provides a preventative barrier that stops age-related brain degeneration. Catechins have special antioxidant properties that protect the cells from death induced by glucose oxidation. Catechins also stop the production of nitric oxide by the glial cells surrounding the neurons. Nitric oxide plays an important role as a neurotransmitter involved in memory formation. But if you have excessive levels, it can lead to neuronal death and neurodegenerative diseases. Flavonoids are very effective in regulating the substances that reduce nitric oxide production in high concentrations. The key is the EGCG.

Over the years researchers have shown a well-recognized connection between an excess of free radicals in the body that are established as oxidative stresses and healthy brain functioning. Research results demonstrate that green tea has particular benefits for promoting healthy brain function by providing antioxidant and EGCG support to brain tissues. As aging occurs, your brain cells are extremely sensitive to free radical attacks. Neurons have low antioxidant content. Your brain's metabolism consumes a large amount of oxygen. Brain cells have a very limited ability to repair damage to their DNA caused by free radicals. Aging causes us to be exposed to a flood of free radicals. This overabundance of free radicals makes it more difficult to maintain healthy brain tissues, but green tea contains antioxidants that help maintain a healthy brain, even as aging occurs. Your brain has the protection of green tea to prevent damage. Green tea promotes healthy communication between your immune system and stranded cells. This process supports the body's natural shielding response to the stressors such as free radicals.

Dr. Anastasis Sephanou of the British Heart Foundation reports that green tea even protects the heart against the damage caused by heart attacks and strokes. A chemical (polyphenols) called EGCG found in green tea reduces cell deaths that lead to tissue death and organ failure. When a person has a heart attack, the amount of oxygen and nutrients reaching the brain and heart is reduced. This leads to cell death and irreversible damage. EGCG speed the recovery of heart cells allowing the tissues to recover and alleviates damage to vital organs.

A study in the February 2006 *American Journal of Clinical Nutrition* investigated the link between green tea and brain health. The results demonstrated that green tea consumption is linked to a reduced prevalence of cognitive impairment. Green tea protects the brain against degenerative processes leading to Alzheimer and Parkinson's diseases. The study results showed that green tea inhibits the buildup of amyloid proteins associated with Alzheimer's. The senior subjects either drank at least two cups of green tea or took 1,000 mg of decaf green tea extract daily. Researchers analyzed data from the 2002 study that involved 1,003 Japanese patients who participated in a comprehensive geriatric assessment. The seniors were aged 70 and up. All completed a special questionnaire that contained questions about their lifestyle, habits, and frequency of green tea consumption. All were evaluated for their cognitive function that measured memory, attention, and language use. The results were very clear. The seniors that consumed green tea or took green tea extract did much better than those that did not. The researchers concluded that green tea has the ability to support brain health. If you cannot drink the 2 cups of green tea daily, take four capsules of green tea extract daily.

The *Journal of Neuroscience* (January 2004) published results of a study about green tea and Alzheimer's. Researchers found a particular ingredient of green tea helps protect the brain against an attack of Alzheimer's disease. The special ingredient is EGCG. EGCG offers protection against certain cancers. The specific information provides evidence that EGCG decreases production of beta-amyloid protein. Beta-amyloid is thought to play a key role in the development of Alzheimer's symptoms and disease. Beta-amyloid is the specific protein that forms the characteristic plaques found in the brain of Alzheimer's patients that is thought to lead to nerve damage and memory loss. Dr. Juan Tan's research findings suggest that a concentrated component of green tea can decrease brain amyloid plaque formation. Green tea certainly has the special nutrients that counter Alzheimer's problem of beta amyloid plaque, and the antioxidants in green tea are key to a healthy brain.

A study by Dr. Kuriyama and colleagues at Tohoku University Medical School showed that drinking green tea reduced cognitive impairments. The lowest risk of impairment was when subjects drank at least two cups daily of green tea. People who drank two cups or more of green tea a day were 54% less likely to have test scores in the cognitive impaired range compared to people who drank a cup of green tea three times a week. People who drank four to six cups of green tea a week were 38% less likely to demonstrate cognitive impairment.

Other research reflects most neuro-degenerative diseases are linked to excessive free radical damage plus an excessive breakdown of neurotransmitters. In the 1998 *Chinese Journal of Physiology*, free radical damage causes continual monoamine oxidase activity (MAO) that contributes to neurological damage that leads to disease. EGCG is effective in inhibiting MAO as well as lowering peroxide levels in glial cells in the brain. Glia cells are nonneuronal cells that supply nutrition and support for homeostasis, form myelin, and facilitate signal communication in the nervous system. Glia cells outnumber neurons in the brain 50 to 1. Some glia cells act as physical support for neurons while others regulate the inner environment of the brain by regulating fluids surrounding neurons and their synapses and providing nourishment for the various nerve cells. Latest research shows the glial cells in the hippocampus and cerebellum actively play a part in synaptic transmission, control clearance of neurotransmitters from synaptic cleft, release of ATP and neurotransmitters.

Green Tea and the Heart

Green tea helps lower cholesterol, blood pressure, and helps prevent atherosclerosis (hardening of the arteries). Dr. Bautista presented a study at the WONCA (World Organization of Family Doctors) in 2004. The study took at 15 patients with elevated cholesterol who were not tea drinkers. The patients were asked to drink a cup of tea three times daily for two weeks. Ten patients finished the study. Total cholesterol dropped from 235 to 187 and LDL (low density lipids) decreased from 144 to 137. Even the blood pressure dropped from an average of 130/87 to 117/81 after the first week and 118/80 after the second. Another clinical trial evaluated the effect of theaflavins enriched green tea on lipids and lipoproteins of patients with mild to moderate hyperlipidemia (elevated blood cholesterol). A double blind, placebo controlled study contained 240 patients, aged 18 years and older on a low fat diet with mild to moderate elevation of blood cholesterol. They were randomly assigned to take a theaflavins-enriched capsule (375 mg) every day or a placebo for 12 weeks. After 12 weeks, LDL-C, HDL-C, and triglycerides decreased while the total cholesterol in the control group did no change remarkably. No major adverse side effect occurred and was well tolerated by the patients. The researchers concluded that green tea is an effective adjunct to reduce LDL-C in patients with high cholesterol.

The May 2002 American Heart Association's journal, *Circulation*, reported that green tea might considerably lower a person's chances of dying from a heart attack. Patients that consumed two or more cups of tea daily had a 44% lower death rate than the patients that did not drink tea. Researchers attribute this to the flavonoid antioxidants naturally present in green tea and by relaxing the blood vessels so blood can flow more easily.

Green Tea and Allergies

The September 2002 *Web MD* reported green tea antioxidants help prevent allergic reactions. Japanese researchers found an ingredient in green tea blocks in allergic reactions and the symptoms that it provokes. EGCG (epigallocatechin gallate) in green tea block the production of two substances that trigger and prolong allergic reactions, histamine and immunoglobulin E (IgE). EGCG affects the mast cells and basophils. These cells cause the release of histamine in allergy sufferers. Hirofumi Tachibana, associate professor of chemistry at Kyushu University in Japan suggests that if you have allergies, you should consider drinking green tea (or taking the green tea extract capsules). For centuries people have used green tea to relieve cold and allergy symptoms such as coughing, sneezing, runny nose and watery eyes.

Green Tea versus Red Wine

For many years links have been made between the effects of green tea and the French people. Researchers found that even though the French eat a diet rich in fat, they had a lower incidence of heart disease that those in the U.S. The answer comes in red wine, which contains resveratrol, a polyphenol that limits the negative effects of smoking and a fatty diet. In 1997 a study done by researchers at the University of Kansas determined that EGCG is twice as powerful as resveratrol. This explains why the rate of heart disease among Japanese men is very low even though approximately 75% are smokers. Since green tea leaves are steamed, it prevents the EGCG compound from being oxidized. The only key is to not drink caffeine. Use decaf green tea or take it in supplement form (decaffeinated green tea extract) 2,000 milligrams (mg) daily. If you smoke, use 3,000 milligrams (mg) daily to protect your heart and lungs. Add Vitamin C (Ester C) and antioxidants for more protection.

Green Tea and Inflammation

Case Western University scientists suggest the green tea antioxidants move blood cells that cause inflammation across the blood vessels walls when green tea is taken on a daily basis. These scientists report that these promising results could create future research that may lead to new arthritis treatments that would help millions. Researchers found that the catechins in green tea lower the toxicity of certain anti-inflammatories, thereby reducing their inflammation causing potential. Inflammation is necessary for healing. When it becomes chronic and causes an inflammatory reaction, then you begin to have problems. Many inflammatory conditions can linger for years and for some, even a lifetime. The end result is internal scarring and chronic degenerative diseases.

Nightshades are a group of plants that often increase inflammation. Nightshades include white potatoes, tomatoes, red and green peppers, pimiento, cayenne peppers, eggplant, and tobacco.   Nightshades frequently exacerbate rheumatic disease and arthritis. Inflammation results from the release of tissue hormones called histamines. High histamine is the last thing you want if you have inflammation and chronic pain. Your key is homeostasis, a total balance of your system. If you cannot give them up, rotate the foods each week so that you are not eating them any more often than every four to five days. For example if you eat tomatoes on Monday, do not each any nightshade in any form until Friday or Saturday. Keep in mind that it may take 2 months to see a change after you discontinue the nightshades to see a difference.

If you have arthritis or fibromyalgia, chronic inflammation can and does occur as a primary event with no preceding period of acute symptoms. In some cases the swelling becomes so severe that you can hardly write. This usually calls for a strong green tea protocol utilizing two capsules, three times daily along with 5,000 mg of Ester C, and two capsules of 400 mg Serrapeptase, three times daily. The 400 mg capsule is the best one to use to assist in the reduction of swelling. Celadrin, a proprietary blend of esterified fatty acid carbons (EFAC) soothes and supports muscle aches and pains, joints, and surrounding tissues. Celadrin reduces inflammation very quickly and is available in a soft gel and a cream. Both work very well. Malic acid also helps detoxify and Boswellia is a natural herbal anti-inflammatory that is safe and effective. Essential fatty acids are a must and you should take two, three times daily for relief. Pay careful attention to your diet. If certain foods such as nightshades cause you to swell more, modify your diet and exclude them from your diet. More inflammation results in more pain, swelling, stiffness, depression, anger, and loss of mobility. Moderate exercise is an excellent tool to help you become more mobile. Remember, it can take up to six weeks for the nightshades to clear your system.

Green Tea & Alternative Health

Studies show that green tea dramatically reduces the risk of many types of cancer including liver, breast, lung, pancreatic, and skin cancers. Researchers think green tea compounds work as a sort of super antioxidant that blocks the interaction of tumor protectors. Green tea and its compounds also lower the risk of heart disease and stroke by preventing the development of blockages in the arteries. Green tea also keeps blood sugars at a healthy low level as well as combat viruses.

Green Tea and Sleep

Researchers from the National Institute of Mental Health in Japan found taking a component of green tea, L-Theanine, produces a major improvement in sleep quality. L-Theanine is an amino acid found in green tea. The clinical study clearly suggests that Suntheanine (L-Theanine) improved the quality of sleep and the mental state upon arising according to Dr. Shuichiro Shirakawa. The subjects fell asleep more quickly and their overall sleep efficiency improved with lifted mood and a decrease in nightmares.

Green Tea and Microbes (Bacteria)

In the April 2004 issue of *Natural Pharmacy,* controlled human studies show that green tea extracts have both preventative and therapeutic effects on dental caries, gastrointestinal (GI) dysbiosis (leaky gut), and chronic gastritis. Dysbiosis or leaky gut is a term for an imbalance and symptoms in the GI tract from alterations in bowel flora. The three major causes of dysbiosis are fungus overgrowth (usually caused by antibiotics with psychological or physical stress), poor diet, and parasites. Symptoms are complex, misleading, and often contribute to many chronic and degenerative diseases. Acute dysbiosis symptoms are diarrhea, nausea, abdominal pain and cramps. Chronic symptoms are loose stool and/or constipation, gas, bloating, food cravings and allergies, fibromyalgia, rheumatoid arthritis, chronic fatigue, and neurological disorders. The intestines exclude microbes from the systemic circulation while absorbing critical nutrients. The intestinal mucosa is exposed to bacterial products, endotoxins, phenols, ammonia, hydrogen sulphides, and indoles that have detrimental effects on the intestines and your body's overall health. Sulfate (mostly derives from food additives) and diets high in protein contribute to production of toxic products. When these byproducts are absorbed, they create a toxic bowel.

In one animal study guinea pigs infected with shigellosis were cured within three days after receiving green tea extract while the control animals died within 24 hours. Laboratory studies show that green tea constituents have significant antibacterial action against E. Coli (the bacterial responsible for fatal outbreaks of gastroenteritis (inflammation of the stomach and GI tract) and hemolytic-uremic (kidney) syndrome after consuming contaminated or undercooked meat. Green tea also inhibits the growth of various bacteria such as cholera and some salmonella that cause diarrhea diseases. Drinking green tea or supplementing with decaf green tea extract could keep you healthy.

Green tea extracts demonstrate bactericidal (agent that destroys bacteria) action of Staphylococcus and Yersinia bacteria and inhibit methicillin-resistant S. aureus (MRSA–antibiotic resistant staphylococcus bacteria that attacks the skin) in vitro. Green tea extracts help make MRSA bacteria less resistant. The data strongly suggests that green tea is a promising vehicle for managing a multitude of infectious conditions, especially the skin and GI tract, and best of all green tea has a high safety record.

Even more research demonstrates that green tea is beneficial with tuberculosis (Mycobacterium tuberculosis or TB). The study found that green tea's EGCG had the ability to down-regulate the gene transcription within human macrophages (type of white blood cells that surround and engulf bacteria). EGCG inhibits TB survival within the macrophages and may play a roll in the prevention of TB infections.

Green Tea and Osteoporosis

Consumption of green tea over many years increases your bone structure and density so that you have less risk of osteoporosis.

The individuals that consumed green tea at least weekly demonstrated improvement in lumbar spine bone density.

Green Tea and Menopause

NIH reports a study conducted in healthy postmenopausal women demonstrated that a twice-daily formula containing green tea effectively reduced menopausal symptoms including hot flashes and sleep disturbances.

Green Tea and Weight

Studies show drinking a cup of tea twice a day before a meals curbs appetite and reduces the formation of excess fat cells. Green tea has thermogenic properties promoting increased heat in the body that burns more calories.

Green Tea and Epilepsy

Some evidence indicates that iron plays a role with epilepsy. Green tea polyphenols inhibit or decrease iron-induced seizures, and decrease the firing of dopaminergic neurons. Since green tea contains theanine, it acts as a mild sedative to the central nervous system.

Green Tea Deodorizing Effects

For centuries it has been know that green tea leaves act as a deodorizer. The Japanese people typically drink green tea with or after a meal. The consumption of green tea neutralizes foul breath (halitosis) that can be generated after garlic, tobacco, fish, onion, etc. The polyphenols are thought to contain the deodorizing agent in green tea. One study of subjects had volunteers gargle with mashed garlic, and then their breaths were collected. Then the subjects ate a green tea candy (3.3 g) that contained 1 mg of green tea extract per gram. After ingesting the candy, their breath, was collected and the halitosis before and after eating the candy was subjected to a sensory test. The scores were graded from 0 to 4 with 0, very strong smell; 1, strong smell; 2, medium smell; 3, weak smell; and 4, no smell. Four panel members examined the subjects and the results were 1.3 with the controls; 3.7 mark after the green tea candy;

and 1.3 after sodium copper chlorophyllin. Green tea positively reduces halitosis so enjoy your cup of tea after dinner.

Green tea diminishes tobacco smoke.

Green Tea Endorsements

Lester Mitscher, Ph.D. of Kansas University and an expert in the causes of cancer was so impressed with studies on green tea that he now takes a daily green tea supplement.

New Anti-Cancer Green Tea Product

Dr. Lee's Tea for Health organic green tea in a bottle is the first green tea in a bottle to meet the *National Cancer Institute's* standard required for anticancer benefits. On July 10, 2006 Dr. Lee presented the new tea and the scientific evidence at the International Union Against Cancer (UICC) quadrennial World Cancer conference in Washington, D.C. The new 710 EGCG organic tea in a bottle is available in four flavors and is the only green tea qualified to make a *FDA approved health claim* regarding the anticancer benefits. The anticancer health benefit of green tea is dose dependent. The minimum anticancer dose is 800 ml of green tea that contains 710 mcg/ml EGCG per day in the adult. This equals two bottles of Dr. Lee's 710 EGCG organic green tea in a bottle.

Brewing Green Tea

More than 3,000 varieties of green tea exist, but they all derive from *Camellia sinensis*. Many factors such as where the tea was grown, the temperature, and how it is dried and processed, and what is added to the tea influence the taste. The most popular green teas include Dragonwell (Lung Ching), Genmai Cha, Gyokuro, Gunpowder, Hojicha, Pi Lo Chin, and Sencha.

Brewing a cup of tea seems simple enough, but use spring or distilled water. Chlorinated water decreases the antioxidant properties of green tea and waters with minerals may change the taste of the tea. Green tea tastes best when you prepare it in water that is cooler than boiling (about 180°F) and allow it to steep for three minutes. If your water is too hot, your tea will taste bitter. If you use loose tea, the proper ratio is one teaspoon of Sencha (Japanese) tea to a cup of water. Use slightly more if you are using Chinese (Pi Lo Chun). If you are using a kettle, water is perfect when it starts to emit a rumbling sound. If you are using a microwave, when the tiny air bubbles begin to form, the water is ready.

The amount of catechins varies from 50 to 100 mg in an average 5 ounce cup of tea. You must drink 3 to 10 cups of green tea to obtain the equivalent of 300 to 1,000 mg of catechins. Taking a decaffeinated green tea extract easily insures that you receive the health benefits without the caffeine. Enjoy your tea!

Bibliography

Adams, Mike. "Green tea phytochemicals shown to prevent breast cancer, colon cancer, lung cancer, and more."www.newstarget.com/0000375.html 12/11/03

Afag, F., N. Ahmad and H. Mukhtar. Suppression of UVB-induced phosphorylation of mitrogen-activated protein kinases and nuclear factor kappa B by green tea polyphenol in SKH-1 hairless mice." *Oncogene.* 2003 December 18: 22(58): 9254-9264.

Almada, Anthony. "Green tea for diabetes." *Delicious* magazine. 2003 March 1.

Anand, P.K., D. Kaul, M. Sharma. "Green tea polyphenol inhibits Mycobacterium tuberculosis survival within human macrophages." *International Journal Biochemistry & Cell Biology.* 2006; 38(4): 600–609.

Anderson, R.A. and M.M. Polansky. "Tea enhances insulin activity." *Journal of Agriculture and Food Chemistry.* 2002; 50: 7182–7186.

Asfar S., S. Abdeen, H. Dashti, M. Khoursheed, H. Al-Sayer, T. Mathew, A. Al-Bader. "Effect of green tea in the prevention and reversal of fasting-induced intestinal mucosal damage." *Nutrition.* 2003 June 19; (6)536–40.

Baliga, M.S., S. Meleth, and S.K. Katiyar. " Growth inhibitory and antimetastatic effect of green tea polyphenols on metastasis—specific mouse mammary carcinoma 4T1 cells in vitro and invivo systems."*Clinical Cancer Research.* 2005 March 1;11(5):1918–1927.

Beauchamp, Kimberly. "Green tea helpful for certain leukemias." *NNFA Today.* 2006 February; 20(2) 6.

"Benefits of green tea: green tea and diabetes." www.imperialteagarden.com/greenteadiabetes.html 7/11/05

Block, Will. "Green tea may help control blood sugar." *Life Enhancement.* www.life-enhancement.com/article_template.asp?ID=794 7/11/05

"Breast cancer and green tea." *Health Bulletin.* www.healthbulletin.org/nutrients/nutrients22.htm. 7/19/06

Brown, Michael D. "Green tea (Camilia sinensis) extract and its possible role in the prevention of cancer." *Alternative Medicine Review.* 1999 October ; 4(5): 360–370.

Bursill, C.A. and P.D. Roach. "Modulation of cholesterol metabolism by the green tea polyphenol (-)-epigallocatechin gallate in cultured human liver (HepG2) cells." *Journal of Agriculture and Food Chemistry.* 2006 Mar 8; 54(5): 1621–1626.

"Can Prostate Cancer Be Prevented?" www.medscape/viewarticle/4984004_print 2/20/05

Chou, Jeyling. "Green tea inhibits cancer growth." *Daily Bruin* online, February 18, 2005.

"Complete Guide to Prostate Health." All About Prostate. http://www.allaboutprostate.com 7/18/06

Cooper, R., D.J. Morre, and D. M. Morre. "Medicinal benefits of green tea: Part I. Review of noncancer health benefits." *Journal of Alternative and Complementary Medicine.* 2005 June: 11(3): 521–528.

"Drinking Tea Linked to Lower Risk of Biliary Tract Cancers and Biliary Stones." *International Journal of Cancer.* 2006; 118:3089–3094.

Dryden, G.W., M. Song, and C. McClain. "Polyphenols and gastrointestinal diseases." *Current Opinions Gastroenterology.* 2006 March; 22(2): 165–170.

Edmonds, Bryce. "Tea makes other supps green with envy." *Natural Foods Merchandiser.* 2005 July 1; XXVI(7): 34, 38.

Esko, Edward, Ed. "A guide to the health benefits of green tea." www.prevmedctr.org/library/lib_greentea_esko.asp 7/19/06

Frances. *Cancer Journal.* 1996 Sept. 9: 161-169

Fujiki H. "Green tea: Health benefits as cancer preventive for humans." *Chemical Record of N.Y.* 2005;5(3):119–132. http://ncbi.nlm.nih.gov/entrez/query.fcgi?db=pubmed&cmd=Retrieve&dopt=Abstract&list_uids=... 7/14/06

Fujiki, Hirota. "Two stages of cancer prevention with green tea." *Journal of Cancer Research and Clinical Oncology.* 1999 October; 125(11): 589–597.

Glial cell. Wikipedia. http://en.wikipedia.org/wiki/glia 5/11/2006

Gao, Y.T., J.K. McLaughlin, W.J. Blot, B.T. Ji, Q. Dai, and J.F. Fraumeni, Jr. "Reduced risk of esophageal cancer associated with green tea consumption. *Journal of National Cancer Institute.* 1994 June 1; 86(11):855–858.

Gilbert, Tom. "Green tea may protect women from breast cancer." 2001 September; www.thedoctorwillseeyounow.com/news/cancer/0901/tea.shtml interMDnet Corp.

Gonzalez de Mejia, E. "The chemo-protector effects of tea and its components." *Archives Latinoam Nutrition. (Archivos latinoamericanos de nutrición).* 2003 June; 53(2):111-118.

Goto, R., H. Masuoka, K. Yoshida, M. Mori, and H. Miyake. "A case control study of cancer of the pancreas." *Gan No Rinsho* (Japanese journal of cancer clinics). 1990 February; Spec. No: 344–350.

"Green tea." University of Maryland. 2004; http://www.umm.edu/altmed/ConsHerbs/Interactions/GreenTeach.html

"Green tea." ACS:Green Tea. (American Cancer Society)www.cancer.org/docroot/ETO/content/ETO/5_3X_Green_Tea.asp?sitearea=ETO 7/19/2006

"Green tea." OncoLink. www.Oncolink.com/search/search.cfm

"Green tea." LHP053. www.gaiaherbs.com

"Green tea and cancer prevention." www.safealternativemedicine,/.co.uk/GreenTeaCancerPrevention.cfm 7/19/06

"Green tea can block cancer." (from *Journal Chemical Research in Toxicology*) *BBC News.* 2003 August 5. www.newsvote.bbc.co.uk/mpapps/pagetools/print/news.bbc.co.uk/2/hi/health/3125469.stm

"Green tea (Camellia sinensis)." MedlinePlus. www.nlm.nih.gov/medline/druginfo/natural/patient-green_tea.html 5/8/06

"Green tea could fight autoimmune disorders." 2006 June 15. http://www.nutraingredients-usa.com/news/ng.asp?id=60691

"Green tea extract can increase endurance by 24 percent and speeds up fat breakdown." www.defeatdiabetes.org/articles/supplements2050209.htm

"Green tea may protect the aging brain." www.forum.lowcarber.org/showthread.php?mode=hybrid&t=287018 6/16/06

"Green tea extract–Green Tea Leaf–Extract Health Benefits." www.bodybuildingforyou.com/health-supplements/green-tea-extract.htm 7/14/06

"Green tea may help explain 'Asian paradox.'" 2006 June 12. www.nlm.nih.gov/medlineplus/news/fullstory_34727.html

"Green tea extract may ward off Alzheimer's." *Nutrition Industry Executive.* 2005 October: 22.

"Green tea—Healthy or Not?" Health 24. 2006 August 6. www.xtramsn.co.nz/news/0,,12078-4471430-117_12535_true,00.html

"Green tea: History and health: Lesson #09." www.teaclass.com/lesson_0209.html. 7/20/06

"Green tea in smoking-related bladder cancer trials." 2004 September 7. www.beveragedaily.com/news/ng.asp?id=53433-green-tea-in

"Green tea lowers diabetes risk, transdermal catechin delivery effective." *Insider.* 2006 May 29: 7.

"Green tea may protect the aging brain." Reuters Feb. 24, 2006 http://www.msnbc.msn.com/id/11547880/#storyContinued

"Green tea shows promise as an allergy fighter." *Prevention.* 2003 April. www.adagio.com/info/health_benefits/news_27.html?SID=711d619bc79aaa0ef6417ef4cb52fece

Greenwald, P. "Clinical trials in cancer prevention: current results and perspectives for the future." *American Journal of Nutrition.* 2004 December;134 (12 Suppl): 3507S–3512S.

Greenwall, Ivy. "Part II. Cardioprotective properties efits of Green Tea." *Life Extension* magazine. 1999 June. www.vivaherbals.com/pages/cardio.html 5/3/06 & 8/20/06

Gruenwalkd, J. T. Brendler, C. Jaenicke. Ed. *PDR for Herbal Medicines.* 2nd ed. Montvale, NJ: Medical Economics Company. 2000: 369–372.

Harby, Karla. "Esophageal adenocarcinoma appears to be affected by common beverages." 2004 May 18 www.medscape.com/viewarticle/478184_print 2/20/05

Harrar, Sari N. "Green tea tackles pollen." *Prevention.* http://www.prevention.com/article/0,5778,s1-3-71-217-2583-1,00.html 8/17/06.

Hawrelak, Jason A. and Stephen P. Myers. "The causes of intestinal dysbiosis: a review." *Alternative Medicine Review.* 2004, June: 9(2):180–197.

Healy, Bernadine. "Green tea and cancer: A mixed bag." *U.S. News & World Report.* 2005, July 14. www.usnews.com/usnews/health/briefs/alternativemedicine/hb050714a.htm 7/19/2006

Heck, A.M., B.A. DeWitt, A.L. Lukes. "Potential interactions between alternative therapies and warfarin." [Review]. *American Journal of Health System Pharmacy.* 2000 July 1; 57(13):1221–1230.

Hibasami, H. T. Komiya, and Y. Achiwa, et al. "Induction of apoptosis in human stomach cancer cells by green tea catechins." *Oncology Reports*. 1998; 5: 527–529.

"How green tea fights cancer and why pregnant women may want to avoid it." *NNFA Today*. 2006 April; 19(4):5.

Hsu, S. "Green tea and the skin." *Journal of the American Academy of Dermatology*. 2006 June; 52(6): 1049–1059.

Hsu, S.D., B.B. Singh, J.B. Lewis, J.L. Borke, D.P. Dickinson, L. Drake, G.B. Caughman, G.S. Schuster. "Chemoprevention of oral cancer by green tea." *General Dentistry*. 2002 Mar-April;50(2):140–146.

Jatoi, A. N. Ellison, P.A. Burch, J.A. Sloan, S.R. Dakhil, P. Novotny, et al. "A phase II trial of green tea in the treatment of patients with androgen independent metastatis prostate carcinoma." *Cancer*. 2003;7(6):1442–1446.

Ji, B.T. W.H. Chow, A.W. Hsing, et al. "Green tea consumption and the risk of pancreatic and colorectal cancers." *International Journal of Cancer*. 1997;70: 255–258.

Ji, B.T, W.H. Chow, A.W. Hsing, J.K. McLaughlin, Q. Dai, Y.T. Gao, W.J. Blot, J.F. Fraumeni, Jr. "Green tea consumption and the risk of pancreatic and colorectal cancers. *International Journal of Cancer*. 1997 January 27; 70(3):255–258. *Journal of Pharmacology,* Vol 58, pp. 599–604, 2006.

Jian, L. L.P. Xie, A.H. Lee and C.W. Binns. "Protective effect of green tea against prostate cancer." *International Journal of Cancer*. 2004;108(1): 130–135.

Joyal, Steven V. "Metabolic Syndrome." *Life Extension* magazine. 2006 July.

Jueneja, L.R. "Trends in Food Science." 1999 June; 10(6/7): 199–204.

Kabuto, H., I. Yokoi, and A. Mori. "Monoamine metabolites, iron induced seizures, and the antioconvulsant effects of tannins." *Neurochemistry Research.* 1992 June; 17(6): 585–590.

Kemberling J.K., J.A. Hampton, R.W. Keck, M.A. Gomez, and S.H. Selman. "Inhibition of bladder tumor growth by the green tea derivative epigallocatechin-3-gallate. *Journal of Urology.* 2003; 170(3): 773–776.

Kono, S., K. Shinchi, K. Wakabayashi, S. Honjo. I. Todoroki, Y. Sakurai, K. Imanishi, H. Nishikawa, S. Ogawa, and M. Katsurada. "Relation of green tea consumption to serum lipids and lipoproteins in Japananes men." *Journal of Epidemiology.* 1996 Sept. 6(3): 128–133.

Koo, M.W. and C.H. Cho. "Pharmacological effects of green tea on the gastrointestinal system. *European Journal of Pharmacology.* 2004 October 1; 500(1–3): 177–185.

Kuo, P.L. and C.C. Lin. "Green tea constituent (-)-epigallocatechin-3-gallate inhibits Hep G2 cell proliferation and induces apoptosis through p53-dependent and Fas-medicated pathways." *Journal of Biomedical Sciences.* 2003 Mar-April;10(2):219–227.

Kuzuhara, T. Y. Sei, K. Yamaguchi, M. Suganuma, and H. Fujiki. "DNA and RNA as new binding targets of green tea catechins." *Journal of Biological Chemistry.* 2006 June 23; 281(25): 17446–17456.

Laifer, Stephen. "The Lancet reports extremely positive data on green tea." *Life Extension* magazine. 2005, January.

Larsson S.C. and A. Wolk. "Tea consumption and ovarian cancer in a population -based cohort." *Archives of Internal Medicine.* 2005 December 12–26; 165(22): 2683–2686.

Lee, M.J., J.D. Lambert, S. Prabhu, X. Meng, H. Lu, P. Maliakal, C.T. Ho, and C.S. Yang. "Delivery of tea polyphenols to the oral cavity by green tea leaves and black tea extract. *Cancer Epidemiology Biomarkers & Prevention.* 2004 January;13(1):132–137.

Lyn-Cook, B.D., T. Rogers, Y. Yan, E.B. Blann, F.F. Kadlubar, G.J. Hammons. "Chemopreventive effects of tea extracts and various components on human pancreatic and prostate tumor cells in vitro." *Nutrition and Cancer.* 1999; 35(1):80–86.

Maiti, T.K. J. Chatterjee, and S. Dasgupta. "Effect of green tea polyphenols on antiogenesis induced by an angiogenin-like protein." *Biochemical and Biophysical Research Communications.* 2003 Aug15: 308 (1):64–67.

Maron, D.J., G.P. Lu, N.S. Cai, Z.G. Wu, Y.H. Li, H. Chen, J.Q. Zhu, X.J. Jin, B.C. Wouters, J. Zhao. "Cholesterol–lowering effect of theaflavin-enriched green tea extract: a randomized controlled trial. *Archives of Internal Medicine.* 2003 June 23; 163(12):1448–1453.

Masuda, M. M. Suzui, J.T. Lim, and I.B. Weinstein. "Epigallocatechin-3-gallate inhibits activation of HER-2/neu and downstream signaling pathways in human head and neck and breast carcinoma cells." *Clinical Cancer Research.* 2003 August 15; 9(9): 3486–3491.

Moss, Ralph W. "What's green, cost pennies, prevents cancer—and, uh, needs more study?" www.ralphmoss.com/html/green.shtml from *The Cancer Chronicles#10* 1991 Autumn. *From The Cancer Chronicles#22* 1993 Autumn.

Mu, L.N. X.F. Zhou, B.G. Ding, R.H. Wang, Z.F. Zhang, C.W. Chen, G.R. Wei, X.M. Zhou, Q.W. Jiang, and X.Z. Yu. "A case-control study on drinking green tea and decreasing risk of cancers in the alimentary canal." Zhonghua Liu Xing Bing Xue ZaZhi (Chinese Journal of Epidemiology). 2003 Mar;24(3): 192–195.

Hawrelak, Jason and Stephen P. Myers. "The causes of intestinal dysbiosis: a review." Alternative Medicine Review. 2004 June; 9(2): 180–197.

Netsch, M.I., H. Gutmann, C.B. Schmidlin, C. Aydogan, and J. Drewe. "Induction of CYP1A by green tea extract in human intestinal cell lines." *Plant Methods.* 2006 May; 72(6): 514–520.

"New Anti-cancer Green Tea Product with FDA Health Claim." www.foodingredientsfirst.com/Newsmaker 7/10/2006.

"New findings on green tea." *Life Extension* Org. www.lef.org/featured-articles/greent.html

"New insight into green tea's action on bladder cancer." www.nowfoods.com/?action=itemdetail&itemid=43568&ref=enews&TPL Name... 2/18/2005

"NIH Funds Trail of Alternative Pancreatic Cancer Therapy." June 8, 2006 www.cancerpage.com/news/article.asp?id=1058.

Norton, Amy. "Early Hope Seen for Green Tea in Fighting Leukemia." 2005 December 21. www.nlm.nih.gov/medlineplus/news/fullstory_28759.html 12/27/2005

Oak, M.N. J. El Bedoui, V.B. Schini-Kerth. "Antiangiogenic properties of natural polyphenols from red wine and green tea. *Journal of Nutritional Biochemistry.* 2005 Jan; 16(1): 1–8.

Oakie, Susan. "Maverick treatment finds U.S. funding." *Washington Post.* Jan. 18, 2000: A01

Oncology Reports, 1998; 5: 527–529.

"Oolong Tea: The Middle Child of the Tea Family." Health Essentials. *NNFA Today.* 2006 July; 20(7)9.

Paajanen, Terri. "Green Tea for Breast Cancer." May 10, 2001 http://coffeetea.about.com/library/weekly/aa100501a.htm 7/19/06

Reeves, Clay. "Green Tea Reduces Prostate Cancer Risk." www.prostatecancer.about.com/od/riskreducers/a/greentea.htm. 7/18/2006.

Roomi, M.W., V. Ivanov, T. Kalinovsky, A. Niedzwiecki, M. Rath. "Antitumor effect of ascorbic acid, lysine, proline, arginine, and green tea extract on bladder cancer cell line MIA PaCa-2. International Journal of Gastrointestinal Cancer. 2005; 35(2): 97–102.

Roomi, M.W., V. Ivanov, T. Kalinovsky, A. Niedzwiecki, M. Rath. "Antitumor effect of ascorbic acid, lysine, proline, arginine, and green tea extract on bladder cancer cell line T-24." *International Journal of Urology.* 2006; 13(4); 415–419.

Sadzuka Y., et al. "Efficacies of tea components on doxorubicin induced antitumor activity and reversal of multi-drug resistance." *Toxicology Letters.* 2000 April3; 114(1–3): 155–162.

Sahley, Billie. *Theanine, The Relaxation Amino Acid.* San Antonio, TX: Pain & Stress Publications. 2004;41–42.

Saleem, M.,V.M. Adhami, I.A. Siddiqui, and H. Mukhtar. "Tea beverage in chemoprevention of prostate cancer: a mini-review. *Nutrition and Cancer.* 2003; 47(1): 13–23.

Sartippour, M.R., R. Pietras, D. C. Marquez-Garban, H.W. Chen, D. Heber, S.M. Henning, G. Sartippour, L. Zhang, M. Lu, O. Weinberg, J.Y. Rao, and M.N. Brooks. "The combination of green tea and tamoxifen is effective against breast cancer." *Carcinogenesis.* 2006 June 19; [Epub ahead of print].

Satoh, E., N. Tohyama, and M. Nishimura. "Comparison of the antioxidant activity of roasted tea with green, oolong, and black teas." *International Journal of Food Science Nutrition.* 2005 December; 56(8): 551–559.

Shetty, M., K. Subbannayya, and P.G. Shivananda. "Antibacterial activity of tea (Camellia sinensis) and coffee (coffee Arabica) with special reference to Salmonella typhimurium." *Journal of Communicable Diseases.* 1994 September; 26(3): 147-150.

Smith, Linda M. "Green Tea Extract Helps Prevent Prostate Cancer." *Life Extension.* 2005 October: 17.

Taylor, Nadine. *Green Tea.* Kensington Publishing Corp. 1998.

"The Story of Green Tea." http://www.linanwindow.com/tea/history.htm

"Smoking: Green tea may protect Asian smokers." *New Zealand Herald.* 2006 June 14. www.subs.nzherald.co.nz/topic/story.cfm?c_id=321&ObjectID=10386427

"Study Shows Green Tea Fights Bladder Cancer." *KSDK News* Channel 5. (NBC News) February 16, 2005.

Sugiyama, T., Y. Sadzuka, K. Tanaka, and T. Sonobe. "Suntheanine shown to enhance the therapeutic efficacy of doxorubicin." *Toxicology Letters.* 2001 April 30; 121(2):89–96.

Sun, C.L, J.M. Yuan, W.P. Koh, and M.C. Yu. "Green tea, black tea and colorectal cancer risk: a meta-analysis of epidemiologic studies." *Carcinogenesis.* 2006 May 2; 27(7): 1301–1309

"Suntheanine for Reducing Stress, Promoting Relaxation, and Improving Quality of Sleep." *Nutrition Industry Executive.* 2006 March;64.

Takada, M., Y. Nakamura, T. Koizumi, T. Kamigaki, H. Toyama, Y. Suzuki, Y. Takeyama, and Y. Kuroda. "Suppression of human pancreatic carcinoma cell growth and invasion by epigallocatechin-3-gallate." *Pancreas.* 2002 July; 25(1): 45–48.

"Tea Constituent Supports Slumber." *Research Report* from Taiyo International . 3/1/2004

'Tea impacts BCI-2 gene: fresh evidence claimed for how tea protects against cancer." 2003 December: www.psa-rising.com/eatingwell/greentea.php. 6/27/05

"Tea Might Protect Transplanted Livers." *Health Daily News.* 2005 February. www.adagio.com/info/health_benefits/news_54.html?SID=711d619bc79aaa0ef6517ef4cb52fece 7/14/06

Thangapazham, R.L., A.K. Singh, A. Sharma, J. Warren, J.P. Gaddipati, R.K. Maheshwari. *Cancer Letter.* 2006 March 3 www.ncbi. nlm.nih.gov/entrez/query.fcgi?db=pubmed& cmd=Retrieve&dopt=Abstract&list_uids... 7/18/2006

"Theaflavins: Green tea and black tea combine a powerful punch against cholesterol." *Advances in Orthomolecular Research.* 2005; Fall: 33–34.

Terashima T., et al. "Effect of Suntheanine intake on learning ability." *Health and Longevity.* 1999 November 18; 82–83.

Toda, M., S. Okubo, R. Ohnishi, and T. Shimamura. "[Antibacterial and bactericidal activities of Japanese green tea.]" *Nippon Saikinaku Zasshi.* 1989 July; 44(4): 669–672.

Vayalil, P.K., C.A. Elmets, and S.K. Katiyar. "Treatment of green tea polyphenols in hydrophilic cream prevents UVB-induced oxidation of lipids and proteins, depletion of antioxidant enzymes and phosphorylation of MAPK proteins in SKH-1 hairless mouse skin." *Carcinogenesis.* 2003 May; 24(5) 927-936.

Vergote, D., C. Cren-Olive, V. Chopin, R.A. Toillon, C.Rolando, H. Hondermarck, X. Le Bourhis. "(-)-Epigallocatechin (EGC) of green tea induces apoptosis of human breast cancer cells but not of their normal counterparts." *Breast Cancer Research Treatments.* 2002 December; 76(3): 195–201.

Weinreb, O., S. Mandel, T. Amit, and M.B. Youdim. "Neurological mechanisms of green tea polyphenols in Alzheimer's and Parkinson's diseases. *Journal of Nutritional Biochemistry.* 2004 Sept; 15(9):506–516.

Whelan, A.M., T.M. Jurgens, and S.K. Bowles. "Natural health products in the prevention and treatment of osteoporosis: systemic review of randomized controlled trials." *Annuals of Pharmacotherapy.* 2006 May; 40(5): 836–849.

Wu, A.H., M.C. Yu, C.C. Tseng, J.J. Hankin, M.C. Pike. "Green tea and risk of breast cancer in Asian Americans." *International Journal of Cancer.* 2003 September 10; 106(4): 574–579.

Wu, A.H., et al. "Green Tea and Soy Linked to Lower Breast Cancer Risk for Asian Americans." *International Journal of Cancer.* 2003 September 10. www.breastcancer.org/green_tea.html 7/19/2006

Wu, A.H., C.C. Tseng, D. Van Den Berg, and M.C. Yu. "Tea intake, COMT genotype, and breast cancer in Asian-American women. *Cancer Research.* 2003 November 1; 63(21):7526–7529.

Yam, T.S., J. M. Hamilton-Miller, S. Shah. "The effect of a component of tea (Camellia sinensis) on methicillin resistance, PBP2 synthesis, and beta-lactamase production in Staphylococcus aureus." *Journal of Antimicrobial Chemotherapy.* 1998 Aug; 42(2): 211–216.

Yamamoto, Takehiko, Lekh Raj Juneja, Chi Djoing-Chi, Mujo Kim, ed. *Chemistry and Applications of Green Tea.* New York: CRC Press, 1997.

Yanagimoto, K. H. Orchi, K.G. Lee, and T. Shibamoto. "Antioxidative activities of volatile extracts from green tea, oolong tea, and black tea."

Journal of Agriculture Food Chemistry. 2003; 51(25):7396–7401).

Yang, T.T., M.W. Koo. "Chinese green tea lowers cholesterol level through an increase in fecal lipid excretion." *Life Science.* 2000; 66(5): 411–423.

Yokogoshi, H., T. Terashima. "Effect of Suntheanine on brain monamines, striatal dopamine release and behavior. *Nutrition.* 2000 September; 16(9): 776–777.

Zhao, X., H. Tian, X. Ma, and L. Li. "Epigallocatechin gallate, the main ingredient of green tea induces apoptosis in breast cancer cells." *Frontiers in Bioscience: A Journal and Virtual Library.* 2006 September 1; 11: 2428–2433.

Index

Addiction in America?
Prescription Medications

For every prescription drug, there is a nutrient that does the same thing in the brain!

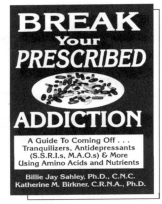

BREAK
Your
PRESCRIBED
ADDICTION

A Guide To Coming Off . . .
Tranquilizers, Antidepressants
(S.S.R.I.s, M.A.O.s) & More
Using Amino Acids and Nutrients

Billie Jay Sahley, Ph.D., C.N.C.
Katherine M. Birkner, C.R.N.A., Ph.D.

- Finally, a step-by-step guide that outlines withdrawal and maintenance from prescription meds or addictive substances.

- Withdrawal schedules and amino acid and nutrient replacement programs included.

- Learn what amino acids and nutrients to use to withdraw safely.

- Answers for your questions regarding medications, natural replacements, and a proven natural approach to recovery.

- Learn why amino acids are so important to your health and by nourishing the brain and body you can successfully withdraw from drugs.

Break Your Prescribed Addiction $14.95

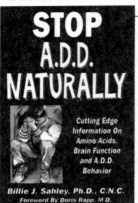
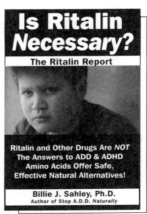

P.T.S.D. & C.E.F.?

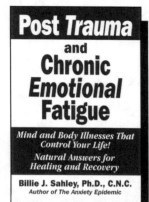

Post Trauma
and
Chronic
Emotional
Fatigue

*Mind and Body Illnesses That
Control Your Life!*

*Natural Answers for
Healing and Recovery*

Billie J. Sahley, Ph.D., C.N.C.
Author of The Anxiety Epidemic

$7.95

Millions of people live their lives in fear, anxiety, and pain. They go from doctor to doctor and do not get answers—they only get drugs!

Post Trauma and Chronic Emotional Fatigue can *control your mind and body.*

This book explains the problems of Post Trauma and Chronic Emotional Fatigue and gives you a complete *natural* treatment plan for healing and recovery.

There is Help for FM?

Over 16 million Americans suffer from Fibromyalgia. This book explores what Fibromyalgia (FM) is and why you have it. Most importantly, it tells you how to get relief from the chronic pain, depression, and feelings of hopelessness.

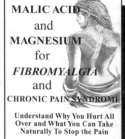

MALIC ACID
and
MAGNESIUM
for
FIBROMYALGIA
and
CHRONIC PAIN SYNDROME

Understand Why You Hurt All
Over and What You Can Take
Naturally To Stop the Pain

Billie J. Sahley, Ph.D., C.N.C.
Author of Break Your Prescribed Addiction

$4.95

A complete *easy-to-follow* program is outlined. Begin to live again *without* pain. The nutritional approach offers hope and relief *without the side effects* experienced with medications. This book gives you *answers* to help your healing process begin, and your constant pain diminishes. There is *natural help for FM.*

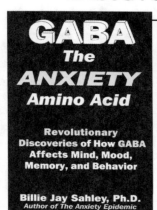
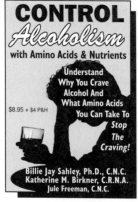

About the Authors

Billie J. Sahley, Ph.D. is Executive Director of the Pain & Stress 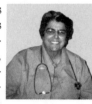 Center in San Antonio. She is a Board Certified Medical Psycho- therapist/Behav- ior Therapist, board certified expert in Trau- matic Stress, and an Orthomo- lecular Therapist specializing in brain chemistry. She is a Diplomate in the American Academy of Pain Management. Dr. Sahley is a graduate of the University of Texas, Clayton University School of Behavioral Medicine, and U.C.L.A. School of Integral Medicine. Additionally, she has studied advanced nutritional biochemistry through Jeffrey Bland, Ph.D., Director of HealthComm. She is a member of the Huxley Foundation/Academy of Orthomolecular Medicine, Academy of Psychosomatic Medicine, North American Nutrition and Preventive Medicine Association. In addition, she holds memberships in the Sports Medicine Foundation, American Mental Health Counselors, and American Academy of Pain Management.

Dr. Sahley has written *The Anxiety Epidemic, Stop A.D.D. Naturally, Chronic Emotional Fatigue, Malic Acid and Magnesium for Fibromyalgia and Chronic Pain Syndrome, The Melatonin Report, GABA, the Anxiety Amino Acid, The Ritalin Report, Theanine, The Relaxation Amino Acid*. She has coauthored *Break Your Prescribed Addiction* and *Heal with Amino Acids*. In addition, she has recorded numerous audio cassette tapes on health related subjects.

Dr. Sahley holds three U.S. patents for Anxiety Control 24, SAF, and Calms Kids (SAF for Kids).

Katherine Birkner is a C.R.N.A., Pain Therapist at the Pain & 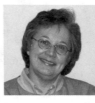 Stress Center in San Antonio. She is a Regis- tered Nurse, Certified Reg- istered Nurse Anesthetist, Ad- vanced Nurse Practitioner, Orthomolecu- lar Therapist, and a Certified Nutritional Con- sultant. She is a Diplomate in American Acad- emy of Pain Management. She attended Brack- enridge Hospital School of Nursing, University of Texas at Austin, Southwest Missouri School of Anesthesia, Southwest Missouri State Univer- sity and Clayton University. She holds degrees in nursing, nutrition, and behavior therapy. Dr. Birkner has done graduate studies through Cen- ter for Integral Medicine and U.C.L.A. Medical School. Additionally, she has studied advanced nutritional biochemistry through Jeffrey Bland, Ph.D., HealthComm. She is a member of The American Association of Nurse Anesthestists and American Academy of Pain Management. She is author of *Break the Sugar Habit Cookbook*, co-au- thor of *Heal with Amino Acids, Control Alcohol- ism, and Break Your Prescribed Addiction*.